On-The-Spot Tips for…

"I GOTTA GO!!!!!!"

(Toilet talk to ease your body, mind, and soul)

Written By
Meagan F. Clements

Copyright © 2023 Meagan F. Clements

Cover art by Des Campbell

All rights reserved. No part of this book may be reproduced, stored, or transmitted by any means—whether auditory, graphic, mechanical, or electronic—without written permission of both publisher and author, except in the case of brief excerpts used in critical articles and reviews. Unauthorized reproduction of any part of this work is illegal and is punishable by law.

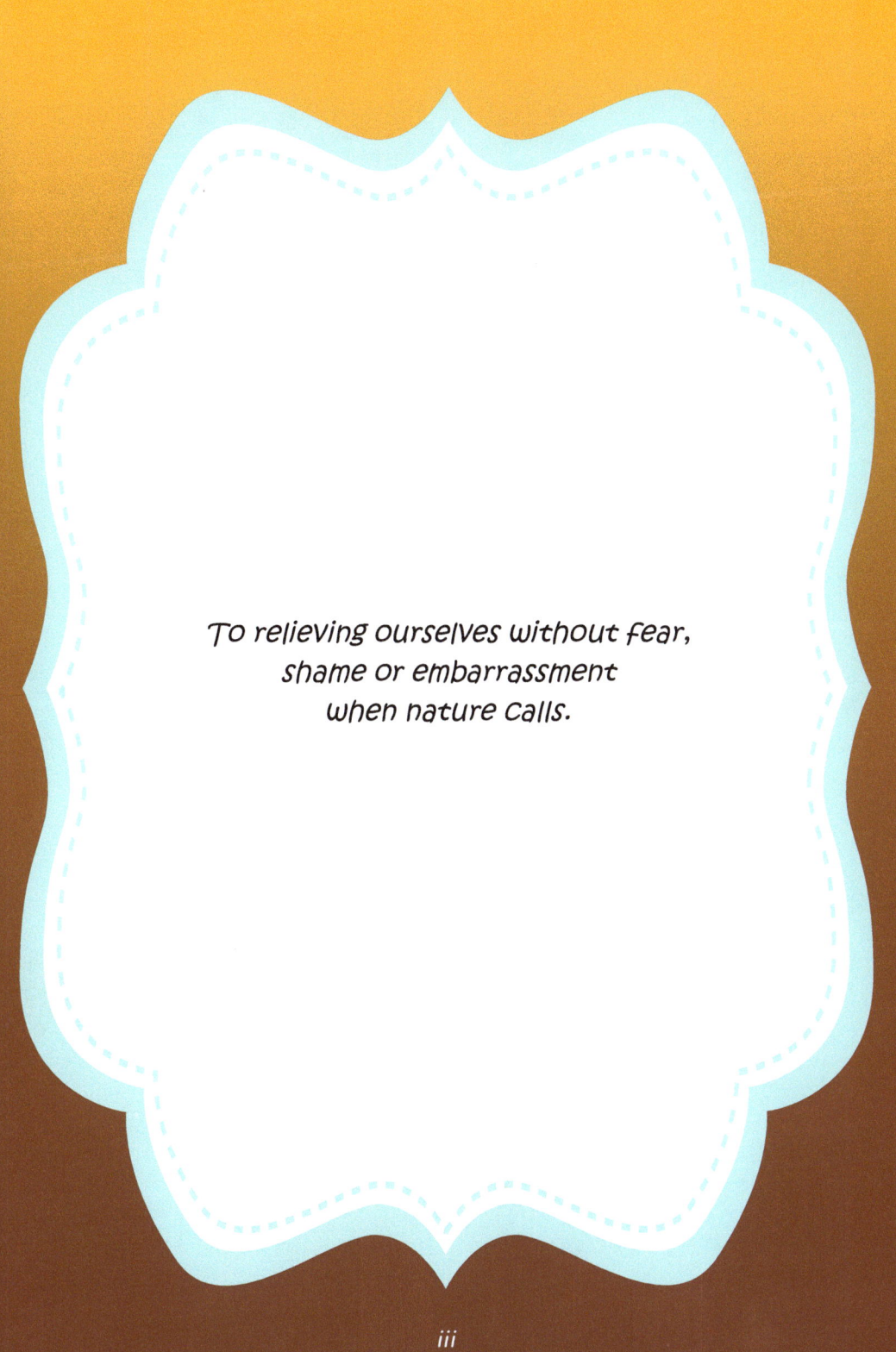

To relieving ourselves without fear,
shame or embarrassment
when nature calls.

Disclaimer

There is no substitute for seeking the advice of a medical professional. If your symptoms persist, speak with your urologist, proctologist, physical therapist, gynecologist, or pelvic floor specialist. A medical professional can assist with issues relative to frequent restroom use.

Tips provided in this book are sprinkled with humor for the enjoyment of the reader. Suggestions provided are based solely upon the author's personal experience.

1

It's only embarrassing if you MAKE it embarrassing. Choose positive mantras over negative self-talk.

Examples:

"I allow myself to use the restroom comfortably and with ease!"

"I love using the restroom!"

"Using the restroom rocks!"

"I can't WAIT to use the restroom again!"

2

Don't be too quick to label yourself. "I have IBS (irritable bowel syndrome)!" or "I suffer from an overactive bladder." Perhaps your symptoms are a direct result of what you ate or drank.

Spicy or acidic foods are common irritants that may increase using the restroom.

Caffeine, alcohol, brown dye, and foods that are rich in potassium such as dried fruit are other common irritants.

Did you know?? White chocolate is better than milk or dark chocolate if you have a sensitive bladder.

Cleaning up your diet prior to an important event, date night, or fun vacation may help your symptoms improve, allowing you to enjoy the time spent with friends, family, or a significant other.

3

Whether you shart or you fart,
Or feel the urge to pee until it
brings you to your knees,
Be proud of who you were created to be.
Own your imperfections like there is no tomorrow,
Dance and celebrate without a need for sorrow!

GLOSSARY

Shart (noun): an instance of accidentally expelling feces when breaking wind.

Shart (verb): expel feces accidentally when breaking wind

4

Reducing stress may reduce using the restroom.

For tips on managing stress in everyday life, purchase On-The-Spot Tips For Reducing Anxiety, Stress, And Nervousness at missmclements.com/additional-books.

Sample <u>tip</u> from the above title:

"Whenever possible, prepare things ahead of time to reduce anxiety the following morning. Prepare a sack lunch, iron what you plan to wear, and take a shower or wash your hair the night before school or work to relieve stress from doing *too* much on the day of."

5

There's no socially acceptable number
of times daily to use the restroom.

Inspector Gadget once said, "Go, go, Gadget go!"

I say, "Go, go, Meagan go!"

You say, "Go, go, [insert your name here] go!"

6

Brainstorm practical solutions for times when you may not be near a restroom.

Long car ride on an open road in the middle of nowhere? No problem! Bring a bottle to relieve yourself in! Keep a roll of toilet paper hidden in your car JUST IN CASE!

Going to the airport where you may get stuck waiting in long lines? Wearing period underwear or a menstrual pad if you are a woman offers protection in case you leak. You may never take advantage of select items; however, knowing you have a layer of protection can provide much needed mental relief.

7

What happened in the past, STAYS in the past. Simply because you had an upset stomach or irritable bladder at an important meeting, during a lunch date with a friend, or at a fancy party, does not mean you should fear doing things in the future. Your symptoms are FLUID and change often from one day to the next.

8

Don't take yourself so seriously. No one else does. When you're in the presence of friends, family, a date, or a significant other and need to relieve yourself often, laugh it off and go with the flow. *pun intended*

9

Don't keep it a secret — chances are, you're experiencing what millions of other people experience EVERY DAY but are afraid to admit. Be brave, be bold, and be an open book. The more open you become about YOUR need to go, the more other people won't have to hide the shame they are feeling about THEIR need to go!

10

Get comfortable with the words poop and potty. Bodily functions are **NORMAL**. Imagine how sick you'd be if you DIDN'T poop or potty.

My adorable Shetland sheepdog, Harmony, loves when I chant, "Go potty! Go potty!" outside.

Each time she goes, she is praised. We need to praise OURSELVES each time we go!

11

Be grateful for the ability to go, treating it as the art form it truly is.

Comedian Daniel Tosh claims there are a wealth of ways to sit on the golden throne, his favorite of which being, reverse or backwards. Have fun with the go!

12

Imagine the toxins you're ridding from your body each time you go.

In a skit featured on *Aged and Confused*, Comedian Bill Engvall claimed he once went SO much poop, he looked down into the great bowl, deep and wide and saw a plastic flamingo!

13

Relax that sphincter muscle! Read, write, draw, or use adult coloring books to help pass the time! There's no such thing as boring when you're in the bathroom!

14

Accidents happen! Relax. It's no big deal. If you think you're the only one who's ever had an accident, you're out of touch with reality. Even pets like Harmony the Shetland Sheepdog have accidents!

15

For years, I worked as a schoolteacher. If you work in an industry where you are unable to go as frequently as you would like and begin to worry, speak with your employer and see what can be done.

Example: get permission for an instructional assistant to watch your students on a field trip while you excuse yourself.

16

If you are in between jobs and looking to get hired by a new company, look for companies that are either a. remote or b. offer more flexibility for you to excuse yourself when needed. TSA officer? Air traffic controller? Theme park ride operator? These jobs might not suit you, given a need to relieve yourself more often.

17

The popular television ad reads, "Got milk?"

Let's rephrase! Got jury duty?

Set up an appointment with your primary care physician, urologist, or even a therapist and express concerns you might have. Perhaps they would consider writing an excuse note on your behalf. A judge likely wouldn't select a juror who is unable sit for longer blocks of time, processing detailed information. This doesn't mean that there's anything wrong with you. Jury duty is simply not the perfect fit.

18

Never stress if your reason for leaving a current job is restroom related. It's perfectly fine if you would prefer switching to a career field allowing more freedom for its employees to use the restroom often. If you gotta go, you gotta go!

19

If people fail at understanding your need to go often (**example:** "You just went five minutes ago!"), that's their problem and not yours. You're only responsible for talking healthy to yourself and loving yourself and your body.

20

Only surround yourself with kind, understanding people who won't make it a big deal every time you have to go. The best friends, family, or significant other are individuals who love you for who you are on the OUTSIDE and INSIDE (and this includes your own bodily functions)!

21

Other people might make assumptions about who you are based on the choices you make in life. Behind your back, they roll their eyes at the term, "remote." As you can probably guess, they view hard working employees as those who work your typical 9 to 5, brief case in hand!

No one is you or lives in your body. You know the truth about you and the choices you've made in life. I'm an author and I work remotely. I also work HARD and diligently.

The perk of my job? I have the freedom to use the restroom when need be. I'll never apologize for that perk or accept other people's assumptions as to WHY I work remotely.

22

Happiness is not reserved for perfect people with perfect bodies. There is no such a thing as a perfect person with a perfect body. No BODY functions perfectly every minute of every second of every day. You deserve to be happy no matter how many times a day you DO or DON'T use the restroom.

23

You body is fluid. It is constantly changing and so is your need to go. How many times you go one day may differ from another and that's OKAY.

24

Learn to accept differences in those you surround yourself with. Not everyone you surround yourself with has a body that functions exactly as yours does. Simply because a friend, family member, date, or significant other DOESN'T use the restroom often, it shouldn't make you feel embarrassed about your own PERSONAL need to excuse yourself for restroom purposes.

25

Everyone has something that they're dealing with. You might stress about the need to go often, but someone else stresses about a different issue. Your issue isn't any worse than what someone else is dealing with.

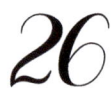

Be careful what you wish for. If you think you'd prefer someone else's struggle over using the restroom often, you'd likely want your own cross back in the end.

27

Don't rule out doing fun stuff with friends or taking exciting trips with family because you're afraid using the restroom often will rear its ugly head. Every major city, theme park, airport, mall, hotel, restaurant, or movie theater has restrooms. PEOPLE will be visiting, and PEOPLE use the restroom!

28

Calm your fears and worries by visiting the website of the vacation destination or other event you are heading to. Scope out where the restrooms are ahead of time! If they don't have info listed on their website, call and speak with a representative. A well-prepared bladder is a happy bladder!

29

Wanna go to that concert or dance club, rocking out to the most awesome music? Does the thought of using the restroom three times in the middle of DJ Fly's smooth moves or Dirty Honey's hour-long set spoil the fun before it's even begun?

Ask the bartender for water in a glass as opposed to a plastic bottle. It looks fancier and you won't feel singled out for being one of the select few without something stylish in hand.

<u>Tip:</u> flavored water is not the same irritant as a sugary drink, but it looks and tastes better than PLAIN water. Pack your favorite flavor pouch in your pocket or purse and stir in the goodness once you arrive. Drink only when you're thirsty and when you do, start with smaller sips. That way, you won't have to relieve yourself as often as someone who is powering their drink at lightning speed.

30

Channel your experiences of using the restroom often into opportunities to affect someone else's life positively. Help someone who may be feeling insecure or embarrassed about THEIR frequent need to go. Channeling something that you once considered a struggle into an opportunity to affect another person's life, takes the pressure and focus off you!

31

Never let your need to use the restroom often stand in the way of your dreams. If your dreams are not bigger than the insecurity you may feel about using the restroom, then you will always be the victim of an upset stomach or sensitive bladder.

32

Bathroom humor is hilarious; however, never take it to the extent of joking about your own issues, making yourself appear weak in the presence of friends, family, or a significant other. Accept what makes you unique without talking down to yourself, even when you are making a joke. Joke about bathroom humor in general without making the joke ABOUT YOU and your personal journey.

33

The algorithm has no guarantee! Ever hear someone say, "You can train your body to use the restroom at select times throughout the day"?

No matter how much you put this theory into practice, you may still need to use the restroom in the middle of attending a play, musical, concert, or while watching a movie at AMC Theaters. Perhaps nature calls while you're on a hike, bike ride, or during a shopping trip at the mall with friends. Simply go with the flow and listen to your body.

34

Be kind to your body. Don't punish it for having to go. The more you make it out to be negative that you're relieving yourself, the more stress and anxiety will build up. As a result, the more you will experience symptoms relative to a touchy tummy or tiny bladder.

35

Understand that your worth and value are not dependent on how many times you DO or DON'T use the restroom on any given day. You're worth it whether you go 6 times or 600 times!

36

Understand that you are not <u>**DEFINED**</u> by how many times you do or don't use the restroom on any given day. Using the restroom three times in an hour might be a piece of your story, but it is certainly not your WHOLE story.

37

Think of all the toilets they sell in kitchen and bath showrooms. Imagine if those toilets could talk. Silly, I know, right? What do you think they would say? Chances are, they would BEG you to purchase them. My point being, it's a toilet's JOB to be used and flushed. Let us give the diverse toilets of the universe a chance to hold number one and number two! Who's with me?!

38

Perhaps you don't use a toilet as a result of a physical disability or temporary medical issue. YOU still matter! Whether you use a catheter, colostomy bag, or both, the feelings of insecurity and embarrassment are still the same. You are still a human being worthy of love and deserve to be treated with dignity and respect.

39

If you are using a catheter and still drive, try a donut-shaped or neck pillow. Also referred to as a hemorrhoid pillow, this practical item may provide additional relief while on the road.

40

Finally, just love. Sometimes the best and most effective thing you can do is to love every toilet you have ever used. Send love to your catheter, colostomy bag, or leak-protectant undergarments. In the words of musician Elton John, "Can YOU feel the love tonight?"

About the Author

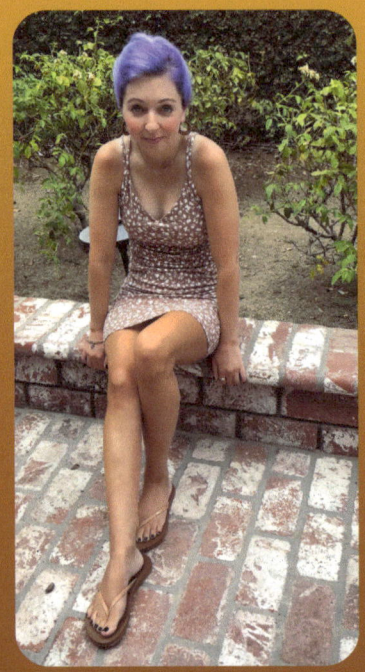

Meagan F. Clements is a credentialed school teacher and writer based in Southern California. She enjoys all aspects of music journalism and creative writing as well as working with children and teens. Her writing stems largely from real life people, events, and experiences.

www.ingramcontent.com/pod-product-compliance
Lightning Source LLC
Chambersburg PA
CBHW040248220526
45473CB00001B/407